The Fat Burning Keto Cookbook

the FAT BURNING keto cookbook

60 delicious ketogenic diet recipes

high fat low carb cooking for lunch & dinner

Recipes365

Copyright © 2017

Recipes365 Cookbooks

All rights reserved. No part of this publication may be reproduced, distributed, or transmitted in any form or by any means, including photocopying, recording, or other electronic or mechanical methods, without the prior written permission of the publisher, except in the case of brief quotations embodied in critical reviews and certain other non-commercial uses permitted by copyright law.

• BEFORE YOU BEGIN •

FREE BONUS GUIDE: TOP 10 KETO DIET MISTAKES

We've put together a free companion guide to go with this recipe book. It features the top 10 mistakes made by people on the ketogenic diet.

If you want to avoid costly mistakes and accelerate your progress you will find a link to the guide at the back of this book. If you can't wait that long, see below now!

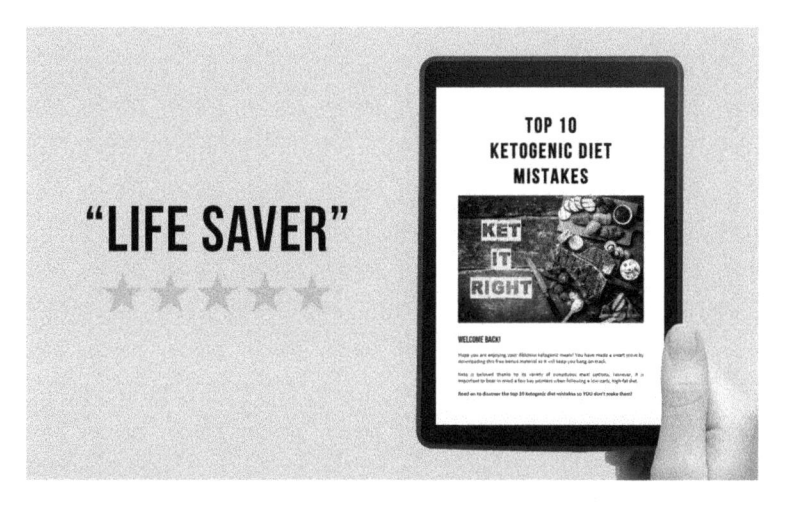

Visit http://geni.us/ketomistakes to get your copy now!

TABLE OF CONTENTS

Introduction 1
   The Science in a Nutshell 1
   What Keto Can do for You 1
   Things to Remember 2

The Recipes 3

Lunches 5
   Keto Flat Bread 6
   Zucchini Boats 7
   Keto Stromboli 8
   Keto Chicken Sandwich 9
   Tuna Bites with Avocado 10
   Keto Green Salad 11
   Original Keto Stuffed Hot Dogs 12
   Easy Egg Soup 13
   Original Nasi Lemak 14
   Keto Sausage and Pepper Soup 15
   Mug Cake with Jalapeño 16
   Fresh Keto Sandwich 17
   Original Squash Lasagna 18
   Chili Soup 19
   Chicken Nuggets for Keto Nuts 20
   Cauliflower Rice with Chicken 21

- Zucchini Keto Wraps 22
- Cauliflower Soup with Bacon and Cheddar 23
- Keto Casserole with Chicken and Bacon 24
- Mexican-Style Casserole with Spinach 25
- Almond Pizza 26
- Chicken Salad 27
- Keto Chicken Thighs 28
- BBQ Chicken Soup 29
- Keto Pork Stew 30
- Keto Enchilada Soup 31
- Grilled Cheese Sandwich 32
- Keto Caprese Salad 33
- Asian Salad 34
- Vegetarian Curry 35

Dinners 37
- Keto Pork Chops 38
- Original Keto Burger with Portobello Bun 39
- Pork Hock 40
- Keto Crisp Pizza 41
- Meatballs with Bacon and Cheese 42
- Bacon Wrapped Chicken 43
- Keto Broccoli Soup 44
- Little Portobello Pizza 45

Bacon Wrap 46

Cheddar Biscuits 47

Sausage & Cabbage Skillet Melt 48

Keto Chicken Tikka Masala 49

Spaghetti Squash with Meat Sauce 50

Keto Guacamole 51

Cheesy Bacon Brussels Sprouts 52

Keto Parmesan Chicken 53

Creamy Chicken 54

Cheeseburger Soup with Bacon 55

Low Carb Chicken Nuggets 56

Keto Salad with Radish and Asparagus 57

Sushi! 58

Kung Pao Chicken 59

Stuffed Burgers 60

Keto Totchos 61

Keto Thai Zoodles 62

Pork Pies 63

Stuffed Peppers 64

Chicken Satay 65

Glazed Salmon 66

Coconut Shrimp 67

INTRODUCTION

Hello there!

Welcome to a wonderful 60 ketogenic lunches and dinners! By now you are probably well aware of the benefits of going keto but just in case you need to refresh your memory, here's a quick top-up before we dive right into the recipes.

THE SCIENCE IN A NUTSHELL

Your body normally converts carbohydrates to glucose for energy. By limiting your intake and replacing it with fats, your body enters a state of ketosis.

Here your body produces ketones, created by a breakdown of fats in the liver. Without carbohydrates as your primary source of energy your body will turn to the ketones instead.

This effectively cranks up the fat burning furnace and puts your body in the ultimate metabolic state.

WHAT KETO CAN DO FOR YOU

Keto has its origins in treating healthcare conditions such as epilepsy, type 2 diabetes, cardiovascular disease, metabolic syndrome, auto-brewery syndrome and high blood pressure but now has much wider application in weight control.

This diet, then, will take you above and beyond typical results and propel you into a new realm of total body health. If you want to look and feel the best you possibly can, all without sacrificing your love of delicious food, then this is the cookbook for you.

THINGS TO REMEMBER

A healthy diet is not solution to anything in and of itself; it must be applied as part of a healthy lifestyle in order to see maximum results.

Think of the ketogenic diet as the foundation of your new body. If you want to build something truly special on top of it then design your lifestyle with that goal in mind.

Cutting out junk food goes without saying, as does ditching bad habits such as smoking and drinking. Exercise, too, will take you to heights you never thought was possible.

So, as you explore these delectable dishes and embark on the keto diet, try not to neglect other areas or responsibility.

Let this be the start of something great!

THE RECIPES

We wanted to make it as simple as possible for you to get in the kitchen and rustle up something special, so you will find each recipe laid out in an easy to follow format.

Each begins with a short intro to the dish, followed by the serving size and list of ingredients. Remember, this diet is designed to rekindle your love of food not extinguish it with rules and regulations, so don't be afraid to experiment.

Use the ingredients as general guidelines and follow the instructions as best you can. You may not get everything perfect first time, every time but that is what makes it yours!

Keep at it for a full 30 days of eating and you will no doubt establish a few firm favorites that you can turn into your specialty dishes over time.

Each recipe ends with a breakdown of key nutritional information including number of calories and amount of fats, carbohydrates and protein.

Again, this isn't to be obsessed over. Food is something to be enjoyed, so if you are going to keep note of your intake levels then just make it a general estimate.

Why no pics? This cookbook is full of *fun* and *flavor*, and doesn't take itself too seriously. The food is entering your mouth, not a modeling contest, and we don't like to encourage unhealthy obsession about presentation. So just cook, experiment, and enjoy.

Once you start loving what you are eating mealtimes will become something to look forward to. Take this as encouragement, go forth and cook to your heart's content!

Lunches

Keto Flat Bread

SERVES 8

For the Crust:

2 cups half-and-half grated mozzarella cheese

2 tbsp. cream cheese

¾ cup almond flour

½ tsp. sea salt

⅛ tsp. dried thyme

For the Topping:

1 cup grated Mexican cheese

½ red onion, small and sliced

4 oz. low carbohydrate sliced ham, cut

¼ medium apple, unpeeled and sliced

⅛ tsp. thyme, dried

Salt and pepper

A classic recipe that will become part of your go-to lunches. This easy recipe has apples, ham and onions – a delicious pizza style combination that you *need* to try!

1. Fill a saucepan with a little water and bring to the boil, then turn the heat to low. Place the saucepan inside a metal mixing bowl to form a double boiler, and add the mozzarella cheese, cream cheese, almond flour, thyme and salt. Stir with a spatula.

2. Cook until the cheese melts, and mix the ingredients into a dough. Pour some onto a 12-inch pizza tray covered with parchment paper. Roll the dough into a ball and place onto the center of the parchment paper. Pat into a disc shape to cover the pan.

3. Place the dough and the parchment paper on the pizza pan, poking holes throughout the dough with a fork, and bake for 6-8 minutes at 425°F. Remove.

4. Spread the toppings over the flatbread, along with the cheese, onion, apple and the ham. Cover with more cheese. Season with thyme, salt and pepper.

5. Bake again at 350°F for 5-7 minutes. Remove once the cheese begins to brown. Let cool before slicing.

NUTRITIONAL INFO PER SERVING

Calories: 257
Fat: 22g
Net Carbs: 5g
Protein: 18g

Zucchini Boats

SERVES 1

2 large zucchini

2 tbsp. butter

3 oz. shredded cheddar cheese

1 cup broccoli

6 oz. shredded rotisserie chicken

1 stalk green onion

2 tbsp. sour cream

Salt and pepper

This stuffed zucchini is an amazing option for a fast and tasty lunch packed with protein.

1. Cut the zucchini in half lengthwise, scooping out the core until you are left with a boat shape.

2. Into each zucchini pour a little melted butter, season and place into the oven at 400°F, baking for about 18 minutes.

3. In a bowl, combine the chicken, broccoli and sour cream.

4. Place the chicken mixture inside the hollowed zucchinis.

5. Top with cheddar cheese and bake for an additional 10-15 minutes.

NUTRITIONAL INFO PER SERVING

Calories: 480

Fat: 35g

Net Carbs: 5g

Protein: 28g

Keto Stromboli

SERVES 4

1¼ cup shredded mozzarella cheese

4 tbsp. almond flour

3 tbsp. coconut flour

1 egg

1 tsp. Italian seasoning

4 oz. ham

4 oz. cheddar cheese

Salt and pepper

Stromboli is a traditional Italian recipe that resembles folded pizza. This keto ham and cheese version is sure to delight.

1. Melt the mozzarella cheese in the microwave for about 1 minute, stirring occasionally so as not to burn it.

2. In a separate bowl, mix almond flour, coconut flour, salt, and pepper and add the melted mozzarella cheese. Mix well. Then, after letting it cool down a bit, add the eggs and combine again.

3. Place the mixture on parchment paper, laying a second layer on top. Using your hands or rolling pin, flatten it out into a rectangle.

4. Remove the top layer of paper and with a knife cut diagonal lines toward the middle of the dough. They should be cut ⅓ of the way in on one side. Then, cut diagonal lines on the other side too.

5. On the top of the dough, alternate slices of ham and cheese. Then, fold one side over, and then the other, to cover the filling.

6. Place on a baking sheet and bake at 400°F for 15-20 minutes.

NUTRITIONAL INFO PER SERVING

Calories: 305

Fat: 22g

Net Carbs: 5g

Protein: 25g

Keto Chicken Sandwich

SERVES 2

For the Bread:

3 eggs

3 oz. cream cheese

⅛ tsp. cream of tartar

Salt

Garlic powder

For the Filling:

1 tbsp. mayonnaise

1 tsp. sriracha

2 slices bacon

3 oz. chicken

2 slices pepper jack cheese

2 grape tomatoes

¼ avocado

Make plain keto cloud bread into a sumptuous chicken sandwich. Bacon and avocado make it even more heavenly.

1. Separate the eggs in different bowls. In the egg whites add cream tartar, salt and beat until stiff peaks form.

2. In another bowl, beat the egg yolks with cream cheese. Incorporate the mixture into the egg white mixture and combine carefully.

3. Place the batter on a parchment paper and form little square shapes that look like bread slices. Sparkle garlic powder on top and bake at 300°F for 25 minutes.

4. While the bread is baking, cook the chicken and bacon in a frying pan, seasoning to taste.

5. When the bread is done, remove from oven and let cool for 10-15 minutes. Then, make the sandwich with the cooked chicken and bacon, adding the mayo, sriracha, tomatoes, cheese and mashed avocado to taste.

NUTRITIONAL INFO PER SERVING

Calories: 360

Fat: 28g

Net Carbs: 3g

Protein: 22g

Tuna Bites with Avocado

SERVES 8

10 oz. drained canned tuna

¼ cup mayo

1 avocado

¼ cup parmesan cheese

⅓ cup almond flour

½ tsp. garlic powder

¼ tsp. onion powder

½ cup coconut oil

Salt and pepper

These unique tuna bites can be served alongside a fresh salad. The avocado packs a fantastic Omega 3 fat punch!

1. In a bowl mix all the ingredients (except coconut oil). Form little balls and cover with almond flour.

2. Fry them in a pan medium heat with melted coconut oil (it has to be hot) until they seem browned on all sides.

NUTRITIONAL INFO PER SERVING

Calories: 137

Fat: 12g

Net Carbs: 10g

Protein: 6g

Keto Green Salad

SERVES 1

2 oz. mixed greens

3 tbsp. roasted pine nuts

2 tbsp. raspberry vinaigrette

2 tbsp. parmesan, shaved

2 slices bacon

Salt and pepper

Who said green salad has to be dull? These ingredients and the heavenly dressing will make your day.

1. Cook the bacon in a pan until crunchy and well browned. Break up into pieces, and add to the rest of the ingredients in a bowl.

2. Dress the salad with the raspberry vinaigrette.

NUTRITIONAL INFO PER SERVING

Calories: 480

Fat: 37g

Net Carbs: 4g

Protein: 17g

Original Keto Stuffed Hot Dogs

SERVES 6

6 hot dogs

12 slices bacon

2 oz. cheddar

½ tsp. cheese garlic powder

½ tsp. onion powder

Salt and pepper

Have just 10 minutes for lunch? No worries, this original recipe is here to help you out!

1. Make a little slit in each hot dog, and stuff them with slices of cheese. Wrap each hot dog with 2 slices of overlapping bacon, and secure with toothpicks.

2. On top of a wire rack (with a cookie sheet below), place the hotdogs. Season them and bake at 400°F for 20-25 minutes approx.

NUTRITIONAL INFO PER SERVING

Calories: 385

Fat: 34g

Net Carbs: 0.5g

Protein: 17g

Easy Egg Soup

SERVES 1

1½ cups chicken broth

½ cube of chicken bouillon

1 tbsp. bacon fat

2 eggs

1 tsp. chili garlic paste

5 minutes and 5 ingredients can make magic stuff—like this yummy egg soup.

1. In a pan on the stove on a medium-high heat, add the chicken broth, bouillon cube and bacon fat. Bring into boil and incorporate chili garlic paste and mix.

2. Whisk the eggs and add them to the chicken while stirring, then let sit for a few minutes.

NUTRITIONAL INFO PER SERVING

Calories: 280

Fat: 25g

Net Carbs: 2.7g

Protein: 13g

Original Nasi Lemak

SERVES 2

For the Chicken & Egg:

2 chicken thighs, boneless

½ tsp. curry powder

¼ tsp. turmeric powder

½ tsp. lime juice

½ tbsp. coconut oil

1 egg

A pinch of salt

For the Nasi Lemak:

3 tbsp. coconut milk

3 slices ginger

½ small shallot

1 cup riced cauliflower

4 slices cucumber

Salt

A food with Indonesian origin, this dish will crown your lunch. It may seem complicated, but it's not too hard; and it will impress, so invite a friend to join you!

1. Rice the cauliflower and strain the water.

2. Prepare the curry powder, turmeric powder, lemon juice and salt, and marinate the chicken thighs for an hour or two in the fridge. Remove and fry.

3. Boil the coconut milk, ginger and shallot in a saucepan. When it bubbles, incorporate the cauliflower rice and mix.

4. Serve with the marinated fried chicken and fried egg.

NUTRITIONAL INFO PER SERVING

Calories: 502

Fat: 40g

Net Carbs: 7g

Protein: 28g

Keto Sausage and Pepper Soup

Serves 6

30 oz. pork sausage

1 tbsp. olive oil

10 oz. raw spinach

1 medium green bell pepper

1 can tomatoes with jalapeños

4 cups beef stock

1 tbsp. onion powder

1 tbsp. chili powder

1 tsp. cumin garlic powder

1 tsp. Italian seasoning

Salt

A delicious low-carb soup that will kill your hunger dead and keep out the cold.

1. In a large pot, heat the olive oil over a medium heat until hot and cook the sausage. Stir.

2. Chop the green pepper and add to the pot. Stir well. Season with salt and pepper. Add the tomatoes and jalapeños. Stir.

3. Add the spinach on top and cover the pot. When it is wilted, incorporate spices and broth and combine.

4. Cover the pot again and let cook for about 30 minutes (heat medium-low). When it is done, remove the lid and let the soup simmer for around 10 minutes.

Nutritional Info per Serving

Calories: 525

Fat: 45g

Net Carbs: 4g

Protein: 28g

Mug Cake with Jalapeño

SERVES 1

2 tbsp. almond flour

1 tbsp. flaxseed meal

1 tbsp. butter

1 tbsp. cream cheese

1 egg

1 bacon slice, cooked

½ jalapeño pepper, sliced

½ tsp. baking powder

¼ tsp. salt

Feeling hot, hot, hot? If you like jalapeño peppers, you'll adore this original mug cake.

1. Cook the bacon on a medium heat in a frying pan until crispy.

2. Mix all the ingredients in a container and pour some inside a mug. Microwave for 75 seconds on high.

3. Carefully take out the mug cake out and let cool before eating.

NUTRITIONAL INFO PER SERVING

Calories: 430

Fat: 40g

Net Carbs: 4g

Protein: 17g

Fresh Keto Sandwich

SERVES 1

1 cucumber

1 ½ oz. boursin cheese

Meat of your choice, sliced

Make this fresh sandwich with ingredients easily found in your fridge. Put into your Tupperware, cover, and go!

1. Slice the cucumber in half and scoop out the core and seeds with a spoon. Remove the hard outer skin carefully with a knife.

2. In one side place cheese. In the other side fold meat. Place together to form a sandwich!

NUTRITIONAL INFO PER SERVING

Calories: 195

Fat: 14g

Net Carbs: 8g

Protein: 18g

Original Squash Lasagna

SERVES 12

1 lb. spaghetti squash

3 lb. ground beef

30 slices mozzarella cheese

1 large jar marinara sauce

32 oz. whole milk ricotta cheese

You've probably used spaghetti squash to make spaghetti. But have you tried it for lasagna?

1. Cut the spaghetti squash in two halves, placing them face down onto a baking dish. Add a half inch or so of water. Bake for 45 minutes. When finished, carefully pull out the meat of the squash.

2. In a frying pan, cook the ground beef the meat in a pan and add marinara sauce.

3. In a greased baking pan, place a layer of spaghetti squash, cover with the meat sauce, mozzarella and ricotta. Repeat until the pan is full.

4. Bake for 35 minutes at 375°F.

NUTRITIONAL INFO PER SERVING

Calories: 710

Fat: 60g

Net Carbs: 17g

Protein: 45g

Chili Soup

SERVES 8

2 tbsp. butter, unsalted

2 onions

1 pepper

8 chicken thighs (boneless)

8 slices of bacon

1 tsp. thyme

1 tsp. salt

1 tsp. pepper

1 tbsp. garlic, minced

1 tbsp. coconut flour

3 tbsp. lemon juice

1 cup chicken stock

¼ cup unsweetened coconut milk

3 tbsp. tomato paste

Use your crockpot to make this yummy soup, perfect for a chilly day. Get it? Good.

1. Place the butter in the center of the Crock-Pot.

2. Slice the onion and pepper, and add to the Crock-Pot. Then add the chicken thighs. Top with the bacon slices.

3. Season with salt, pepper, minced garlic, and coconut flour. Add the lemon juice, chicken stocks, coconut milk and tomato paste.

4. Cook on low for 6 hours. When it is done, stir and serve.

NUTRITIONAL INFO PER SERVING

Calories: 395

Fat: 20g

Net Carbs: 8g

Protein: 40g

Chicken Nuggets for Keto Nuts

SERVES 4

1 chicken breast, precooked

½ ounce grated parmesan

2 tbsp. almond flour

½ tsp. baking powder

1 egg

1 tbsp. water

These are quick, and healthier than any nuggets you'll ever buy off the shelf! Try them and see for yourself.

1. Cut the chicken breast into slices and then into bite size pieces. Set aside.

2. Combine the parmesan, almond flour, baking powder, and water. Stir.

3. Cover the chicken pieces into the batter, and then place directly into the hot oil. Remove when golden.

NUTRITIONAL INFO PER SERVING

Calories: 165

Fat: 9g

Net Carbs: 3g

Protein: 25g

Cauliflower Rice with Chicken

SERVES 6

4 chicken breasts

1 packet curry paste

1 cup water

3 tbsp. ghee

½ cup heavy cream

1 head cauliflower

Riced cauliflower is a good option when you have to cook for a lot of people. Also, it is low-carb, and when combined with curry chicken, you'll have a great source of protein.

1. In a large pan, melt the ghee, add the curry, and stir. When combined, add the water, and simmer for 5 minutes.

2. Add the chicken, cover and keep cooking for 20 minutes more. When it is done, add the cream and cook for 5 additional minutes.

3. Separately, prepare the cauliflower rice: chop the head into florets and shred. Sauté in a frying pan with a little butter or olive oil, and then turn to low, covering with a lid. Let it steam for 5-8 minutes.

4. Serve along with the chicken curry.

NUTRITIONAL INFO PER SERVING

Calories: 350

Fat: 16g

Net Carbs: 10g

Protein: 40g

Zucchini Keto Wraps

SERVES 6

1 zucchini

6 oz. soft goat's cheese

1 tbsp. dried mint

1 tsp. dried dill

Salt and pepper

Oil

This one has to be tried to be believed. It serves up to 6 and the mixture of goat's cheese, mint and dill give it a totally unique twist.

1. Cut off the ends of the zucchini. Slice into ⅛-inch slices and brush with oil. Grill on both sides.

2. Mix together the goat's cheese, mint and dill. Divide into 6 pieces.

3. Wrap the cheese pieces with the zucchini slices and secure with a toothpick.

NUTRITIONAL INFO PER SERVING

Calories: 188

Fat: 14g

Net Carbs: 4g

Protein: 15g

Cauliflower Soup with Bacon and Cheddar

SERVES 6

1 head of cauliflower

2 tbsp. olive oil

1 medium onion, diced

4 slices bacon

1 tbsp. minced garlic

1 tsp. thyme

12 oz. aged cheddar

1 oz. parmesan cheese

3 cups chicken broth

¼ cup heavy cream

This soup will warm you up on a cold day. The hearty bacon and cheddar flavor makes it one that even picky eaters will gobble right up!

1. Chop the cauliflower, and place on a foil-lined baking sheet. Sprinkle olive oil and season it with salt and pepper. Bake for 35 minutes at 375°F.

2. In a pot, cook the bacon until crispy. Add diced onion and fry it in the bacon grease. When it is tender, add the garlic and the thyme, and cook for 1 minute or less.

3. Incorporate the chicken broth and cauliflower, and simmer, covered, for 20 minutes.

4. Once time is up, blend the ingredients in a food processor or blender until smooth. Place back into the pot. Add the cheddar and the parmesan cheese, and stir until melted.

5. Finally, add the bacon and the double cream, and mix well. If needed, simmer for 10 minutes more, or until heated.

NUTRITIONAL INFO PER SERVING

Calories: 340
Fat: 26g
Net Carbs: 10g
Protein: 20g

Keto Casserole with Chicken and Bacon

SERVES 12

12 chicken thighs

1 small onion

4 celery stalks

24 oz. Jimmy Dean sausage

16 oz. sliced mushrooms

16 oz. frozen cauliflower

7 slices bacon

8 oz. shredded cheddar cheese

16 oz. cream cheese, softened

Paprika

This casserole is a complete meal: chicken, bacon, sausage, veggies and cheese will help you stay full of energy for the rest of your day.

1. In the oven, cook the bacon at 400°F for 15 minutes.

2. Meanwhile, dice the chicken and cook in a frying pan. Remove from pan.

3. Brown the sausage. Once it is done, transfer it to the same bowl as the chicken.

4. Chop the onion and celery, and cook them in the remaining sausage grease until translucent.

5. Defrost the cauliflower, and cut the florets into smaller pieces.

6. In a large bowl, add all the ingredients and mix well. Add the cream cheese and mix well.

7. In large pan, place the mixture and sprinkle the paprika.

8. Bake at 350°F for 30 minutes, covered with a foil. Uncover and cook for an additional 10 minutes.

NUTRITIONAL INFO PER SERVING

Calories: 600

Fat: 41g

Net Carbs: 6g

Protein: 53g

Mexican-Style Casserole with Spinach

SERVES 12

1 green pepper

1 onion

20 oz. drained spinach

2 lb. ground pork

2 cans drained diced tomatoes with green chilies

10 tbsp. sour cream

8 oz. mozzarella cheese, shredded

16 oz. cream cheese

4 tsp. taco seasoning

Jalapeños, sliced

This low-carb casserole has all the yummy flavor of tacos, but with a healthier twist.

1. Chop pepper and onion and cook them until translucent. Optional: add diced jalapeños.

2. Place the pepper and onion into a bowl.

3. Cook the spinach by wilting it in a frying pan with a little olive oil. When it is done, add it to the bowl.

4. Cook the ground pork until browned. Season with taco seasoning.

5. Add the diced tomato to the bowl, and incorporate the sour cream, mozzarella and cream cheese. Pour the mixture into a baking dish, and bake at 350°F for 40 minutes.

NUTRITIONAL INFO PER SERVING

Calories: 400

Fat: 30g

Net Carbs: 10g

Protein: 25g

Almond Pizza

SERVES 4

¾ cup almond meal

1½ tsp. baking powder

1½ tsp. granulated sweetener

½ tsp. oregano

¼ tsp. thyme

½ tsp. garlic powder

2 eggs

5 tbsp. butter

½ cup alfredo sauce

4 oz. cheddar cheese

Pizza can be a healthy option when you make the crust with almond meal. Add your favorite toppings and enjoy.

1. Mix the dry ingredients together in a large bowl.

2. Take the eggs (at room temperature) and add to the dry mixture.

3. Melt the butter and incorporate.

4. On a greased pizza pan, spread the crust and pre-cook at 350°F for about 7 minutes.

5. Remove from the oven, and spread the Alfredo Sauce and cheddar cheese on top. Let cook for 5 minutes more.

NUTRITIONAL INFO PER SERVING

Calories: 460

Fat: 45g

Net Carbs: 5g

Protein: 15g

Chicken Salad

SERVES 6

4 chicken breasts

1½ cups cream

4½ oz. celery

4 oz. green peppers

1 ounce green onions

¾ cup sugar free sweet relish

¾ cup mayo

3 eggs, hard-boiled

Fresh and nutritious, this easy recipe can be part of a whole meal or served as a side.

1. Place the chicken in an oven-safe pan, and cover it with cream. Cook for 40-60 minutes at 350°F. When it is done, let cool. Discard the liquid.

2. Chop the celery, pepper and onions, and combine them in a bowl. Dice the chicken and add too.

3. Add chopped hardboiled eggs and mix gently.

3. Divide into 6 containers.

NUTRITIONAL INFO PER SERVING

Calories: 415

Fat: 24g

Net Carbs: 4g

Protein: 40g

Keto Chicken Thighs

SERVES 6

16 chicken thighs (boneless skinless)

2 cups water

8 oz. cheddar cheese, shredded

24 oz. spinach

Salt and pepper

Garlic powder

Three main ingredients. Thirty minutes. One delicious dinner. You can also divide into containers for a yummy lunch option!

1. Bake the chicken thighs in a covered pan with 2 cups of water at 350°F for 20 minutes. Remove and let cool.

2. Break the chicken into pieces, adding the spinach, cheese, and seasonings.

NUTRITIONAL INFO PER SERVING

Calories: 390

Fat: 25g

Net Carbs: 4g

Protein: 47g

BBQ Chicken Soup

SERVES 4

3 medium chicken thighs
2 tsp. chili seasoning
2 tbsp. olive oil
1½ cups chicken broth
1½ cups beef broth
BBQ sauce
¼ cup reduced sugar ketchup
¼ cup tomato paste
2 tbsp. Dijon mustard
1 tbsp. soy sauce
1 tbsp. hot sauce
2½ tsp. liquid smoke
1 tsp. Worcestershire sauce
1½ tsp. garlic powder
1 tsp. onion powder
1 tsp. chili powder
1 tsp. red chili flakes
1 tsp. cumin
¼ cup butter
Salt and pepper

A low-carb soup that comes with an original BBQ flavor. A surefire winner every lunchtime.

1. Take the chicken thighs and de-bone. Reserve the bones. Season with favorite chili seasoning. Bake for 50 minutes at 400°F on a baking tray with foil.

2. In a pot, place olive oil and set on medium high heat. Once it is hot, add the chicken bones. Cook them for 5 minutes and add the broth. Season with salt and pepper.

3. When chicken is done, take off the skin. Incorporate the fat from the chicken into the broth and stir.

4. Make the BBQ Sauce: combine all the already mentioned ingredients for the sauce. Add it to the pot and stir. Let it simmer 20-30 minutes.

5. Emulsify all the fats and liquid together with an immersion blender. Shred the chicken and incorporate into the soup. Cook for 10-20 minutes more.

NUTRITIONAL INFO PER SERVING

Calories: 490

Fat: 38g

Net Carbs: 4.5g

Protein: 25g

Keto Pork Stew

SERVES 4

1 lb. pork shoulder, cooked and sliced

2 tsp. chili powder

2 tsp. cumin

1 tsp. garlic, minced

½ tsp. salt

½ tsp. pepper

1 tsp. paprika

1 tsp. oregano

¼ tsp. cinnamon

2 bay leaves

6 oz. button mushrooms

½ jalapeño, sliced

½ onion, medium

½ sliced green bell pepper

½ sliced red bell pepper

Juice of ½ a lime

2 cups gelatinous bone broth

2 cups chicken broth

½ cup strong coffee

¼ cup tomato paste

This stew is perfect for when the rain is drizzling down the window outside, and you the family fancies a little pick-me-up.

1. Dice the vegetables, and sauté them in a pan lined with olive oil over high heat. Remove from heat when browned.

2. Chop pork and put into a slow cooker with mushrooms, bone broth, chicken broth and coffee.

3. Incorporate spices and vegetables as well and mix. Place the lid. Cook for 4-10 hours on low.

NUTRITIONAL INFO PER SERVING

Calories: 385

Fat: 29g

Net Carbs: 6.4g

Protein: 20g

Keto Enchilada Soup

SERVES 4

3 tbsp. olive oil

3 diced celery stalks

1 medium diced red bell pepper

2 tsp. minced garlic

1 cup diced tomatoes

2 tsp. cumin

1 tsp. oregano

1 tsp. chili powder

½ tsp. cayenne pepper

½ cup chopped cilantro

4 cups chicken broth

8 oz. cream cheese

6 oz. shredded chicken

Juice of ½ a lime

This soup is both spicy and creamy, and so delicious that you'll forget all about how healthy it is.

1. In a hot pan with olive oil, sauté the celery and pepper. When the celery starts to become tender, add the tomatoes and cook for 2-3 minutes longer.

2. Incorporate the spices. Add the chicken broth and cilantro, letting it boil. Reduce to a low heat, and simmer for about 20 minutes.

3. Add the cheese and boil again. Reduce to a low heat and simmer for 25 minutes more.

4. Add the shredded chicken with the lime juice. Stir.

5. Season with cilantro and serve.

NUTRITIONAL INFO PER SERVING

Calories: 345

Fat: 31g

Net Carbs: 6.3g

Protein: 13g

Grilled Cheese Sandwich

Serves 1

2 eggs

2 tbsp. almond flour

1 ½ tbsp. psyllium husk powder

½ tsp. baking powder

2 tbsp. soft butter

2 oz. cheddar cheese

1 tbsp. butter

A crispy option for lunch, and even better with soup on the side, this little number will have you drooling.

1. Mix the eggs, almond flour, psyllium husk powder, baking powder and butter to make the bun. It should be very thick. Place the mixture into a square container and let it sit to level itself. Microwave for 90 seconds.

2. When it is cooked, remove and slice in half. Place the cheese between the bun, and fry in a pan with melted butter over a medium heat.

Nutritional Info per Serving

Calories: 794

Fat: 72g

Net Carbs: 5g

Protein: 30g

Keto Caprese Salad

SERVES 1

1 tomato

6 oz. fresh mozzarella cheese

¼ cup chopped fresh basil

3 tbsp. olive oil

Freshly cracked black pepper

Salt

This simple recipe takes a quick 5 minutes, but is chock-full of fresh flavor.

1. Put the fresh basil in a food processor with some oil. Blend until it forms a paste.

2. Slice the tomatoes and chop the mozzarella. On the top of each tomato, lay the mozzarella and basil paste. Season with olive oil, black pepper and salt.

NUTRITIONAL INFO PER SERVING

Calories: 407

Fat: 38g

Net Carbs: 3.7g

Protein: 16g

Asian Salad

SERVES 1

1 packet shirataki noodles

2 tbsp. coconut oil

1 cucumber

1 spring onion

¼ tbsp. red pepper flakes

1 tbsp. sesame oil

1 tbsp. rice vinegar

1 tsp. sesame seeds

Salt and pepper

Cucumbers are the fresh tasting stars of this dish. Includes the crunch of fried shirataki noodles, and a slightly spicy flavoring to make it more interesting.

1. Wash the shirataki noodles. Strain off all the excess water. Let them dry on a paper towel.

2. In a pan, heat the coconut oil over a medium-high, and fry the noodles for 5-7 minutes. Remove and set on a paper towel to cool.

3. Peel and slice the cucumber. Arrange on a plate, and add the rest of the ingredients, sprinkling over the cucumber. Let chill for 30 minutes in the fridge.

4. Top with fried shirataki noodles.

NUTRITIONAL INFO PER SERVING

Calories: 418

Fat: 45g

Net Carbs: 8g

Protein: 3g

Vegetarian Curry

SERVES 2

4 tbsp. coconut oil

¼ onion, chopped

1 tsp. garlic, minced

1 cup broccoli florets

Spinach

1 tbsp. red curry paste

½ cup coconut cream (or coconut milk)

2 tsp. soy sauce

1 tsp. ginger

2 tsp. fish sauce

This red curry combines unique flavors and leaves you with an easy recipe that your taste buds will love!

1. On a medium-high heat, add the coconut oil to a pan. Once it is hot, sauté the onions until browned. Add the garlic. Turn to a medium-low heat and add the broccoli. Stir.

2. Once the broccoli is partially cooked, add the curry paste. Let it cook for 1 minute.

3. Add the spinach. When it is cooked, add coconut cream and coconut oil.

3. Mix and add the soy sauce, ginger and fish sauce. Simmer for approximately 10 minutes.

NUTRITIONAL INFO PER SERVING

Calories: 395

Fat: 40g

Net Carbs: 7g

Protein: 6g

Dinners

Keto Pork Chops

SERVES 4

½ tsp. peppercorns

1 medium star anise

1 stalk lemongrass

4 halved garlic cloves

4 pork chops (boneless)

1 tbsp. fish sauce

1 tbsp. almond flour

1½ tsp. soy sauce

1 tsp. sesame oil

½ tsp. five spice

½ tbsp. sambal chili paste

½ tbsp. sugar free ketchup

A delicious Asian dinner option with a sumptuous sweet and spicy sauce. This one is guaranteed to be a winner on weekends.

1. Pulverize the peppercorn and star anise (using blender or a mortar).

2. Mix the lemongrass with garlic, fish sauce, soy sauce, sesame oil and five spice powder. Add the powdered peppercorn and star anise. Blend in a food processor until combined.

3. Set the pork on a tray and cover with the mixture on both sides. Cover the tray and marinate for 1-2 hours.

4. Lightly cover each pork chop with almond flour, and pan-fry them at a high temperature. Sear the outsides. Make sure they are done on both sides.

5. Remove and chop into strips.

6. Mix the sambal chili paste and sugar-free ketchup to make the dipping sauce, and serve.

NUTRITIONAL INFO PER SERVING

Calories: 224
Fat: 10g
Net Carbs: 5g
Protein: 35g

Original Keto Burger with Portobello Bun

SERVES 1

2 Portobello mushroom caps

½ tbsp. organic extra virgin coconut oil

1 garlic clove

1 tbsp. oregano

6 oz. organic grass fed beef or bison

1 tbsp. Dijon mustard

1 tsp. salt

1 tsp. freshly ground black pepper

¼ cup cheddar cheese

Salt and pepper

Reimagine the burger by knocking up this awesome recipe and enjoy without shame!

1. Clean the Portobello mushrooms, removing the stems and scraping the gills.

2. In a bowl, combine coconut oil with garlic, oregano, salt and pepper. Marinade the Portobello mushrooms in the mixture while you complete the other steps.

3. In a separate bowl, combine the ground meat, mustard, salt, black pepper and cheddar cheese. Form the patties.

4. Place the mushroom caps on a grill for 7-10 minutes. Remove and cook the burgers for 6 minutes on each side.

5. Remove both from the heat and assemble the burger. Add preferred toppings and serve.

NUTRITIONAL INFO PER SERVING

Calories: 730

Fat: 50g

Net Carbs: 5g

Protein: 60g

Pork Hock

SERVES 2

1 lb. pork hock

¼ cup rice vinegar

⅓ cup soy sauce

⅓ cup shaoxing cooking wine

¼ cup sweetener

⅓ onion

1 tbsp. butter

Shiitake mushrooms

1 tsp. Chinese five-spice

1 tsp. oregano

2 crushed garlic cloves

A Chinese style recipe. It has all the nutrients needed for your keto diet and will be a frequent dinner on your table.

1. Fry the onions in a frying pan until semi-transparent. Meanwhile, boil the mushrooms until tender.

2. In a third pan, sear the pork hock until browned on all sides.

3. After a few minutes, add all the ingredients in a Crock-Pot and cook for 2 hours on a high heat. Stir, then cook for 2 further hours.

4. Remove the pork and bone it. Slice it and put it back to the pot so that it absorbs more flavor.

5. Serve with the vegetables.

NUTRITIONAL INFO PER SERVING

Calories: 550

Fat: 32g

Net Carbs: 20g

Protein: 50g

Keto Crisp Pizza

Serves 12

8 oz. package of cream cheese (at room temperature)

¼ cup parmesan cheese, grated

2 eggs

1 tsp. garlic powder

½ lb. ground beef

1 chorizo sausage

½ tsp. cumin

¼ tsp. basil

½ tsp. Italian seasoning

¼ tsp. turmeric

Salt and pepper

A low-carb option that can be served either hot or cold and big enough to feed the whole family!

1. Mix cream cheese, parmesan cheese, eggs, pepper and garlic with a hand blender.

2. Grease a baking pan with butter. Spread the dough mixture evenly inside. Cook for 12-15 minutes on the oven at 375°F.

3. Cook the meat in a frying pan and add the spices: cumin, basil, Italian seasoning and turmeric.

4. Once the pizza crust is done, let it cool for 10 minutes, and then cover with tomato sauce and some cheese. Bake for 10 minutes more, and when the cheese starts to melt, add the meat. Broil for 5 minutes more. When it is done, let it cool and slice it up.

NUTRITIONAL INFO PER SERVING

Calories: 145

Fat: 12g

Net Carbs: 1g

Protein: 9g

Meatballs with Bacon and Cheese

SERVES 5

1½ lb. ground beef

¾ cup pork rinds, crushed

¾ tsp. salt

¾ tsp. pepper

¾ tsp. cumin

¾ tsp. garlic powder

¾ cup cheddar cheese

4 slices bacon

1 egg

Take meatballs to the next level. These are juicy and taste great. An especially awesome option when you have people over!

1. Process the pork rinds to make a powder.

2. Mix the ground beef, pork rinds, salt, pepper, cumin and garlic powder. Add the cheese and mix well.

3. Cut the bacon into small pieces and fry them in a hot pan until they reach the desired doneness. Let them cool. Add the bacon to the meat and combine well.

4. Form the meatballs.

3. Cook the meatballs in a pan, browning them on all sides, then cover with a lid for 10 minutes. When finished, let them sit for 5 minutes or so before enjoying. Top with the sauce of your choice.

NUTRITIONAL INFO PER SERVING

Calories: 450

Fat: 26g

Net Carbs: 3g

Protein: 50g

Bacon Wrapped Chicken

SERVES 4

2 skinless chicken breasts, boneless

2 oz. blue cheese

4 slices ham

8 slices bacon

A simple recipe with chicken and bacon, sure to go down as a winner in everyone's book. It's easy to make it and absolutely stacked with protein.

1. Slice the breast halves in half lengthwise.

2. Lay out 2 slices of ham, and place a line of cheese in the middle. Roll up, and place inside the chicken breast.

3. Wrap the chicken breast with 4 slices of bacon, covering the entire breast.

4. Place the breasts in an oven-proof skillet (greased with butter or coconut oil), and brown the bacon all over. Remove from the skillet and place in the oven to cook for 45 minutes at 325°F. Let sit for 10 minutes before serving.

NUTRITIONAL INFO PER SERVING

Calories: 270

Fat: 11g

Net Carbs: 0.50g

Protein: 38g

Keto Broccoli Soup

SERVES 4

1 head broccoli

¼ cup heavy cream

¼ cup cream cheese

¼ cup sour cream

¼ cup almond milk

4 oz. cheddar cheese

½ onion

½ chicken bouillon cube

You can probably find all the ingredients for this one in your fridge already, so knock it up and enjoy!

1. Remove the florets from the broccoli. Steam them on the stove.

2. Put the florets into a blender and add the rest of the ingredients. Blend until the mixture reaches the desired consistency.

3. Pour into a pot and simmer until heated (10 minutes or so).

NUTRITIONAL INFO PER SERVING

Calories: 270

Fat: 25g

Net Carbs: 8g

Protein: 10g

Little Portobello Pizza

SERVES 1

3 Portobello mushrooms

Olive oil

3 tsp. pizza seasoning

3 tomato slices

9 spinach leaves

1½ oz. mozzarella

1½ oz. Monterey jack

1½ oz. cheddar cheese

12 pepperoni slices

These little pizzas are made from Portobello caps. An original way to finish your day and keep those cravings in check.

1. Prepare the Portobello mushrooms by washing them, removing both the gills and the stems.

2. Sprinkle with olive oil and pizza seasoning, and then top with all the other ingredients, except the pepperoni slices.

3. Cook at 450°F for 6 minutes. Add the pepperoni slices and broil until crispy.

NUTRITIONAL INFO PER SERVING

Calories: 275

Fat: 20g

Net Carbs: 5g

Protein: 20g

Bacon Wrap

SERVES 4

16 oz. beef

Montreal steak seasoning

4 bacon slices

Delicious, packed with protein and ready to roll nice and fast. What's not to love?

1. Cut the beef into cubes and season it.

2. Cut the bacon slices in four.

3. Wrap the beef with the bacon, and pierce with a toothpick. Repeat 2 or 3 times. Fry for 3 minutes.

NUTRITIONAL INFO PER SERVING

Calories: 217

Fat: 10g

Net Carbs: 0g

Protein: 30g

Cheddar Biscuits

SERVES 1

2 cups Carbquik

2 oz. unsalted butter, cold

4 oz. shredded cheddar cheese

½ tsp. garlic powder

½ tsp. salt

¼ cup heavy cream

¼ cup water

We adore our cheddar biscuits. Stuff them with your favorite fillings, or have them as a side to your favorite dinner dish.

1. In a bowl, mix Carbquik and add the cold butter. Cut in the pieces of butter until the mixture has little balls of butter and flour about the size of peas. Add the cheese, garlic powder and salt and combine together.

2. Add the heavy cream and water. Mix until a dough forms. Separate them into 6 pieces and place on a greased sheet. Bake them at 450°F for about 8-10 minutes.

NUTRITIONAL INFO PER SERVING

Calories: 45

Fat: 4g

Net Carbs: 2.5g

Protein: 1.6g

Sausage & Cabbage Skillet Melt

SERVES 4

4 spicy Italian chicken sausages

1½ cups green cabbage, shredded

1½ cups purple cabbage, shredded

½ cup onion, diced

2 tsp. coconut oil

2 slices Colby jack cheese

2 tsp. fresh cilantro, chopped

Mildly spicy, super satisfying and perfect for a keto dinner. Try this one out with company.

1. Shred the cabbage (or use pre-shredded cabbage) and chop the onion.

2. Melt the coconut oil, and fry the onion and cabbage in a large skillet. Turn to medium-high and cook for 8 minutes.

3. Add the sausage, and stir to mix it into the vegetables. Cook for 8 further minutes.

4. Add the cheese on top and cover.

5. Turn off the heat and wait while the cheese melts into the vegetables.

NUTRITIONAL INFO PER SERVING

Calories: 233

Fat: 15g

Net Carbs: 5g

Protein: 20g

Keto Chicken Tikka Masala

SERVES 5

1 lb. chicken thighs (boneless/skinless)

2 tbsp. olive oil

2 tsp. onion powder

3 minced garlic cloves

1 inch grated ginger root

3 tbsp. tomato paste

5 tsp. garam masala

2 tsp. smoked paprika

4 tsp. kosher salt

10 oz. diced tomatoes (can)

1 cup heavy cream

1 cup coconut milk

Fresh chopped cilantro

1 tsp. guar gum

Chicken Tikka Masala is a super flavorful and delicious curry that you can now make keto style!

1. De-bone the chicken thighs. Chop the chicken into bite-sized pieces.

2. In a slow cooker, add the chicken and grate the ginger on top.

3. In another bowl, mix the tomato paste and canned tomatoes with the rest of the dry spices. Add ½ cup coconut milk and stir. Add to the slow cooker.

3. Cook on low for 6 hours or on high for 3 hours.

4. Once finished, add the remaining coconut milk, double cream, and guar gum. Mix.

NUTRITIONAL INFO PER SERVING

Calories: 495

Fat: 43g

Net Carbs: 5g

Protein: 25g

Spaghetti Squash with Meat Sauce

SERVES 8

2 spaghetti squashes

2 lb. ground beef

33-oz. jar of spaghetti sauce

1 tbsp. minced garlic

1 tbsp. Italian seasoning

Parmesan cheese

It's not even funny how easy this is - and it's just as good as the real thing!

1. Cut the spaghetti squash in half and scrape out the guts. Cook the remaining shell and meat in a glass container partially filled with water at 375°F for 45 minutes or until soft.

2. Brown some beef on the stove. Add the seasonings, the sauce, and mix. Heat through.

3. Carefully remove the cooked spaghetti squash from the oven, and use a fork to create the spaghetti. Serve with the sauce.

NUTRITIONAL INFO PER SERVING

Calories: 170

Fat: 15g

Net Carbs: 12g

Protein: 11g

Keto Guacamole

SERVES 8

4 avocados

1 small onion, chopped

2 tomatoes, chopped

1 jalapeño, chopped

1 tbsp. lime juice

½ tsp. salt

½ tsp. cumin

½ tsp. salt

½ tsp. cayenne pepper

1 tbsp. minced garlic

No recipe book is compete without guacamole, and we've got the perfect keto mix right here.

1. In a large bowl, add the chopped and peeled avocados and the lime juice. Mash the avocados with a potato masher and add spices.

2. Add the jalapeños, onions and tomatoes and mix again.

3. Let rest for an hour before serving.

NUTRITIONAL INFO PER SERVING

Calories: 141

Fat: 11g

Net Carbs: 12g

Protein: 4g

Cheesy Bacon Brussels Sprouts

SERVES 4

5 slices bacon

16 oz. Brussels sprouts

6 oz. cheddar cheese

The combination of cheese and bacon transform this much maligned vegetable into everybody's new best friend!

1. Fry the bacon until crisp. Cut into small pieces.

2. Shred the Brussels sprouts with a food processor. In the bacon grease, fry them until tender.

3. Add in the bacon and cheese when the Brussels sprouts are crispy and translucent.

4. Cook until melted.

NUTRITIONAL INFO PER SERVING

Calories: 260

Fat: 22g

Net Carbs: 5g

Protein: 17g

Keto Parmesan Chicken

SERVES 4

For the Chicken:
3 chicken breasts
1 cup mozzarella cheese
Salt and pepper

For the Coating:
2½ oz. pork rinds
¼ cup flaxseed meal
½ cup parmesan cheese
1 tsp. oregano
½ tsp. salt
½ tsp. pepper
¼ tsp. red pepper flakes
½ tsp. garlic
2 tsp. paprika
1 egg
1½ tsp. chicken broth

The Sauce
¼ cup olive oil
1 cup tomato sauce
½ tsp. garlic
½ tsp. oregano
Salt and pepper

A keto twist on the traditional Italian dish that will make your mouth water and your stomach purr with satisfaction.

1. In a food processor, grind up the pork rinds, parmesan cheese and spices.

2. Slice the chicken breasts into thirds, and season them with salt and pepper.

3. In another bowl, make the coating: whisk eggs and add the chicken broth.

4. Begin to make the sauce by combining all the sauce ingredients in a saucepan and whisking. Let simmer for 20 minutes.

5. Bread the chicken slices: dip them into the egg mixture and then into the pork rind coating. Place on a piece of foil.

6. In a pan, heat a few tbsp. of olive oil and fry the chicken. Place the fried chicken into a casserole dish, cover with sauce and cheese. Bake for 10 minutes at 400ñF.

NUTRITIONAL INFO PER SERVING

Calories: 646
Fat: 47g
Net Carbs: 5g
Protein: 49g

Creamy Chicken

SERVES 1

5 oz. chicken breast

1 tbsp. olive oil

3 oz. mushrooms

¼ small onion, sliced

½ cup chicken broth

¼ cup heavy cream

½ tsp. dried tarragon

1 tsp. grain mustard

Salt and pepper

A unique recipe that will make a special dinner. Chicken is always a good source of fats and proteins.

1. Cut the chicken into cubes, season them, and brown with olive oil. Remove and place on a plate.

2. Add mushrooms to the same pan and cook until browned. Add the onion and cook until the onion is translucent.

3. Add the chicken broth. Reduce by letting it boil for 3-5 minutes.

4. Add the rest of the ingredients and seasonings, and mix. Add the chicken, and let it simmer 3-5 more minutes.

NUTRITIONAL INFO PER SERVING

Calories: 489

Fat: 43g

Net Carbs: 5g

Protein: 30g

Cheeseburger Soup with Bacon

SERVES 5

5 slices bacon

12 oz. ground beef

2 tbsp. butter

3 cups beef broth

½ tsp. garlic powder

½ tsp. onion powder

2 tsp. brown mustard

½ tsp. red pepper flakes

1 tsp. chili powder

1 tsp. cumin

2½ tsp. tomato paste

1 medium dill pickle, diced

1 cup shredded cheddar cheese

3 ounce cream cheese

½ cup heavy cream

1½ tsp. salt

½ tsp. black pepper

Cheeseburger soup? With bacon? Yeah, you're just going to have to trust us on this one.

1. Cook the bacon in a frying pan until crispy. Remove and crumble into a small bowl.

2. In the leftover bacon fat, brown the ground beef.

3. Transfer the meat into a soup pot, adding both butter and spices. Let the butter melt.

4. Incorporate beef broth, tomato paste, cheese and pickles and cook until melted. Cover the pot, turn to low heat and simmer for 20 minutes more.

5. Turn the stove off, and add the double cream and crumbled bacon. Mix well.

NUTRITIONAL INFO PER SERVING

Calories: 573

Fat: 48g

Net Carbs: 4g

Protein: 24g

Low Carb Chicken Nuggets

SERVES 4

For the Nuggets:

24 oz. chicken thighs

1 egg

For the Crust:

1½ oz. pork rinds

¼ cup flax meal

¼ cup almond meal

Zest of 1 lime

⅛ tsp. garlic powder

¼ tsp. paprika

¼ tsp. chili powder

⅛ tsp. onion powder

⅛ tsp. cayenne pepper

¼ tsp. salt

¼ tsp. pepper

For the Sauce:

½ cup mayonnaise

½ avocado

¼ tsp. garlic powder

1 tbsp. lime juice

⅛ tsp. cumin

½ tsp. red chili flakes

This is a different take on the traditional nugget, but you may just end up loving it even more.

1. Dry the chicken and cut into bite-size pieces.

2. Put all the crust ingredients into a food processor and mix.

3. In a bowl place the crumbs and a whisked egg in a different one. Dip the chicken into the egg, the crust and then lay on a greased baking sheet. Bake for 15-20 minutes at 400°F.

4. To make the sauce, just mix all the sauce ingredients together.

NUTRITIONAL INFO PER SERVING

Calories: 615

Fat: 53g

Net Carbs: 2g

Protein: 39g

Keto Salad with Radish and Asparagus

SERVES 4

1½ lb. asparagus spears

10 radishes

4 oz. sour cream

1 tbsp. lemon juice

1 tsp. white wine vinegar

1 tbsp. dill

1 tbsp. mayonnaise

1 tbsp. olive oil

1 tsp. parsley

Pepper

This salad goes well with your favorite grilled chicken, fish or meat, but it can also make a whole meal by itself if you're feeling light and fresh.

1. Boil the water in a pot with a dash of salt. Wash the asparagus stalks and cut off the woody ends. Add to the pot and boil for 2-3 minutes or until desired softness.

2. Place the asparagus into a pot of ice water to stop the cooking process.

3. Cut the tops and bottoms off the radishes and slice them thinly.

4. Make the dressing by blending the rest of the ingredients.

5. Mix the dressing, radishes, and asparagus together until evenly coated.

NUTRITIONAL INFO PER SERVING

Calories: 156

Fat: 10g

Net Carbs: 10g

Protein: 5g

Sushi!

SERVES 3

16 oz. cauliflower

6 oz. softened cream cheese

1-2 tbsp. unseasoned rice vinegar

1 tbsp. soy sauce

5 sheets nori

1-½-inch length of cucumber

½ avocado

5 oz. smoked salmon

You won't believe it: sushi for your keto diet! Here is a simple recipe you can use for movie nights with family and friends.

1. Rice the cauliflower with a food processor.

2. Cut each cucumber into thin lengthwise slices. Keep in the fridge until ready.

3. Cook the cauliflower rice in a hot pan until almost tender. Season with soy sauce. When it is done, mix in a bowl with cream cheese and rice vinegar, and set in the fridge until cool.

4. Thinly slice the avocado.

5. Place a nori sheet on a bamboo roller. Spread some of the cauliflower over the nori sheet to almost cover. Layer the cucumber, avocado and salmon on one end. Roll tightly.

NUTRITIONAL INFO PER SERVING

Calories: 350

Fat: 26g

Net Carbs: 6g

Protein: 18g

Kung Pao Chicken

SERVES 3

For the Chicken:

2 medium chicken thighs

1 tsp. ground ginger

¼ cup peanuts

½ green pepper

4 de-seeded red bird's eye chilies

2 large spring onions

Salt and pepper

For the Sauce:

1 tbsp. soy sauce

2 tbsp. chili garlic paste

2 tsp. rice wine vinegar

1 tbsp. reduced-sugar ketchup

½ tsp. maple extract

2 tsp. sesame oil

10 drops liquid stevia

Asian food for dinner is always a great option. This dish tastes amazing and is super easy to make. The combination of peanuts and chicken give it a keto kick.

1. Cut the chicken into small pieces and season with salt, pepper and ginger.

2. Cook the chicken in a pan over a medium-high heat until browned (approximately 10 minutes).

3. Make the sauce by combining all the sauce ingredients.

4. Chop the vegetables and chilies. When the chicken is done, add all the ingredients and cook for 3-4 minutes longer. Add the sauce and let it boil until reduced.

NUTRITIONAL INFO PER SERVING

Calories: 360

Fat: 27.5g

Net Carbs: 3g

Protein: 22g

Stuffed Burgers

SERVES 2

8 oz. ground beef

1 tsp. salt

½ tsp. pepper

1 tsp. Cajun seasoning

1 ounce mozzarella cheese

2 oz. cheddar cheese

1 tbsp. butter

2 slices pre-cooked bacon

These stuffed burgers are so delicious. You can make them on the grill, or even in the oven if the weather isn't on your side.

1. Take the ground beef and season it with salt, pepper and Cajun seasoning. Flatten into a patty and place mozzarella cheese inside. Cover and flatten again.

2. In a pan, heat the butter (1 tbsp. per burger). Then add the burger, cooking for 2-3 minutes on each side. Top with cheese, cover with a lid and let steam for 2 minutes more.

3. Slice the bacon slices in half and place on top.

NUTRITIONAL INFO PER SERVING

Calories: 615

Fat: 50g

Net Carbs: 1.5g

Protein: 35g

Keto Totchos

SERVES 2

2 servings keto tater tots

6 oz. ground beef

2 oz. shredded cheddar cheese

2 tbsp. sour cream

6 sliced black olives

1 tbsp. salsa

½ jalapeño pepper, sliced

Totchos are crisp tater tots dressed like nachos and topped with sour cream, salsa and jalapeños. Using keto tater tots, this recipe will fulfill your every craving.

1. In a small casserole pan, place 9-10 keto tots and add half of the ground beef and half of the cheese. Place a second layer of tots, and add the rest of the meat and cheese.

2. Broil in the oven for 5 minutes until the cheese melts, and serve with sour cream, black olives, salsa and jalapeño.

NUTRITIONAL INFO PER SERVING

Calories: 638

Fat: 53g

Net Carbs: 6g

Protein: 32g

Keto Thai Zoodles

SERVES 1

3½ oz. chicken thighs

½ tsp. curry powder

3½ oz. zucchini

1 stalk spring onion

1 clove garlic

1 tsp. soy sauce

½ tsp. oyster sauce

⅛ tsp. white pepper

1 tbsp. butter

1 tbsp. coconut oil

1 egg

1⅕ oz. bean sprouts

1 tsp. lime juice

Chopped red chilies

Salt and pepper

A dish all the way from Asia is now available on your dinner table in keto form!

1. Marinate the chicken with curry powder, salt and pepper.

2. Make the zoodles out of the zucchini by slicing it into very thin strips. Chop the onion and garlic into small pieces.

3. Make the sauce by mixing the soy sauce, oyster sauce and white pepper.

4. Cook the chicken with the butter until they are browned and cut into bit-sized pieces.

5. In the same pan on high heat, add coconut oil and sauté the onion and the garlic. Add the egg and cook until slightly browned.

6. Add in the bean sprouts and zoodles, and mix. Pour in the sauce, add the chicken, and stir.

7. Garnish with some chopped red chillies and lemon juice.

NUTRITIONAL INFO PER SERVING

Calories: 581

Fat: 50g

Net Carbs: 7g

Protein: 26g

Pork Pies

SERVES 4

1 lb. ground pork

4 tbsp. grated parmesan cheese

2 beaten eggs

½ tsp. ground nutmeg

½ tsp. ginger

½ tsp. cardamom

½ lemon zest

4 tart shells (keto)

Salt and pepper

This amazing recipe with Irish roots is a great dinner choice when you need something simple and hearty.

1. In a pan over a high heat, place the meat and spices. When it is slightly cooked, remove and add the egg and lemon.

2. Put some of the mixture into keto pie shells and bake for about 20-25 minutes. Remove from oven and let cool.

NUTRITIONAL INFO PER SERVING

Calories: 560

Fat: 23g

Net Carbs: 6g

Protein: 30g

Stuffed Peppers

SERVES 1

4 poblano peppers

1 lb. ground pork

1 tbsp. bacon fat

1 tsp. cumin

1 tsp. chili powder

½ onion

1 tomato

7 baby bella mushrooms

¼ cup packed cilantro

Salt and pepper

This easy recipe includes a delicious combination of vegetables, mushrooms and pork. Stuffed pepper never tasted so good!

1. In the oven, broil the poblano peppers for approximately 8-10 minutes.

2. Brown the pork in bacon fat. Season with salt, pepper, cumin and chili.

3. Incorporate the diced onion and minced garlic. Mix everything together and add the sliced mushrooms. Once they absorb all the fat in the pan, add the chopped cilantro and tomato. Cook for 12 minutes.

4. Put the mixture into the peppers, and bake for 8 minutes at 350°F.

NUTRITIONAL INFO PER SERVING

Calories: 368

Fat: 27g

Net Carbs: 6g

Protein: 22g

Chicken Satay

SERVES 3

1 lb. ground chicken

4 tbsp. soy sauce

3 tbsp. peanut butter

1 tbsp. erythritol

1 tbsp. rice vinegar

2 tsp. sesame oil

2 tsp. chili paste

1 tsp. minced garlic

¼ tsp. cayenne

¼ tsp. paprika

½ tsp. lime juice

2 chopped spring onions

⅓ sliced yellow pepper

This is a low-carb dish that is easy, tasty, and different. Your whole family will love it.

1. In a pan over a medium-high heat, put the sesame oil and sauté the ground chicken. Add the rest of the ingredients and mix well.

2. When it is cooked, add the onions and yellow pepper, mix, and enjoy.

NUTRITIONAL INFO PER SERVING

Calories: 395

Fat: 24g

Net Carbs: 4g

Protein: 35g

Glazed Salmon

SERVES 2

10 oz. salmon filet

2 tbsp. soy sauce

2 tsp. sesame oil

1 tbsp. rice vinegar

1 tsp. ginger, minced

2 tsp. garlic minced

1 tbsp. red boat fish sauce

1 tbsp. sugar free ketchup

2 tbsp. white wine

Salmon is an excellent source of Omega 3 fats, which are key in your keto diet. You'll enjoy this one just as much as your body does.

1. In a container, add all the ingredients (except for the ketchup, sesame oil and white wine) and marinate the salmon in them for 10-15 minutes.

2. In a pan over high heat bring add sesame oil to smoke point and place the filet in, skin side down.

3. Cook until crisp on both sides (4 minutes per side). Remove the fish to make the glaze.

4. Add ketchup and white wine to the marinade. Put in the pan and simmer for 5 minutes, or until reduced to a glaze.

NUTRITIONAL INFO PER SERVING

Calories: 372

Fat: 24g

Net Carbs: 3g

Protein: 35g

Coconut Shrimp

SERVES 3

For the Coconut Shrimp:

1 lb. peeled and de-veined shrimp

2 egg whites

1 cup unsweetened coconut flakes

2 tbsp. coconut flour

For the Sweet Chili Dipping Sauce:

½ cup sugar free apricot preserves

1 ½ tsp. rice wine vinegar

1 tbsp. lime juice

1 medium diced red chili

¼ tsp. red pepper flakes

A traditional recipe turned low-carb. And don't worry, it's still crispy and delicious!

1. Beat the egg whites until they form soft peaks. Prepare two separate bowls with coconut flakes and coconut flour.

2. Dip the shrimp and in coconut flour, then egg whites, and then coconut flakes. Place the shrimp onto a greased baking sheet. Bake at 400°F for 15 minutes. Flip and broil for 3-5 minutes, or until browned and crispy.

3. Make the sauce by mixing all the ingredients for the dipping sauce.

NUTRITIONAL INFO PER SERVING

Calories: 398

Fat: 22g

Net Carbs: 7g

Protein: 36g

FREE BONUS GUIDE:
Top 10 Keto Diet Mistakes

We hope you enjoy making your way through the delicious meals contained in this cookbook, and want to offer you a little something extra to ensure you stay safe and maximize your results.

With our free bonus guide you will learn the top 10 mistakes people make when cooking keto, and discover exactly how to avoid them for yourself. Curious? Use the link below to see it now!

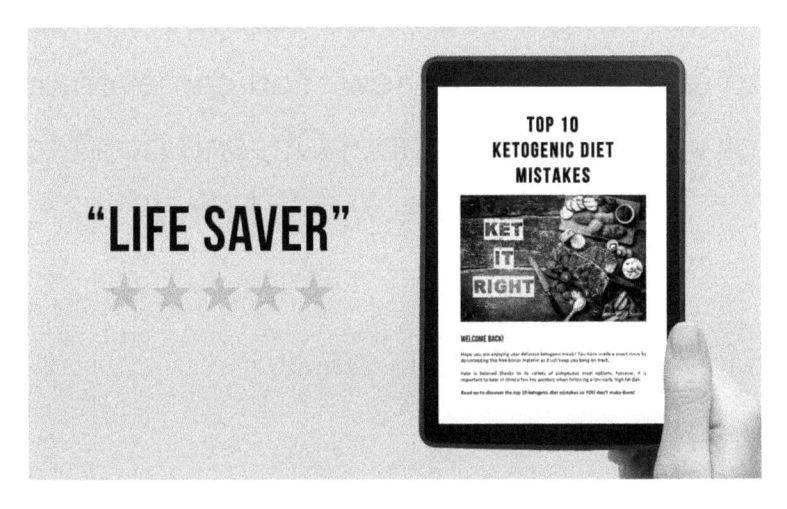

Visit **http://geni.us/ketomistakes** to get your copy now!

Like This Book?

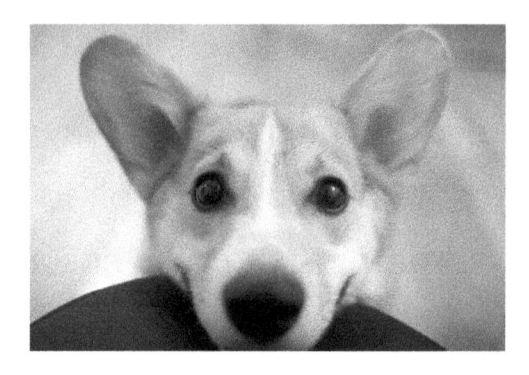

This is Buster, and he'd really love to know what you thought!

If you got value from this book, or the free bonus guide, it would be amazing if you could visit your Amazon order history to leave a quick review. You can even upload a picture of your favorite recipe! Oh, and don't forget to share the love with a friend!

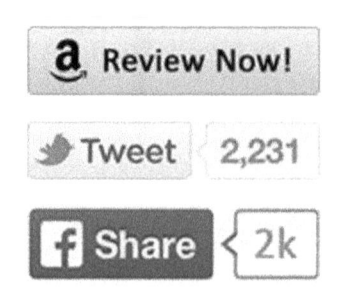

a Review Now!

Tweet 2,231

f Share 2k

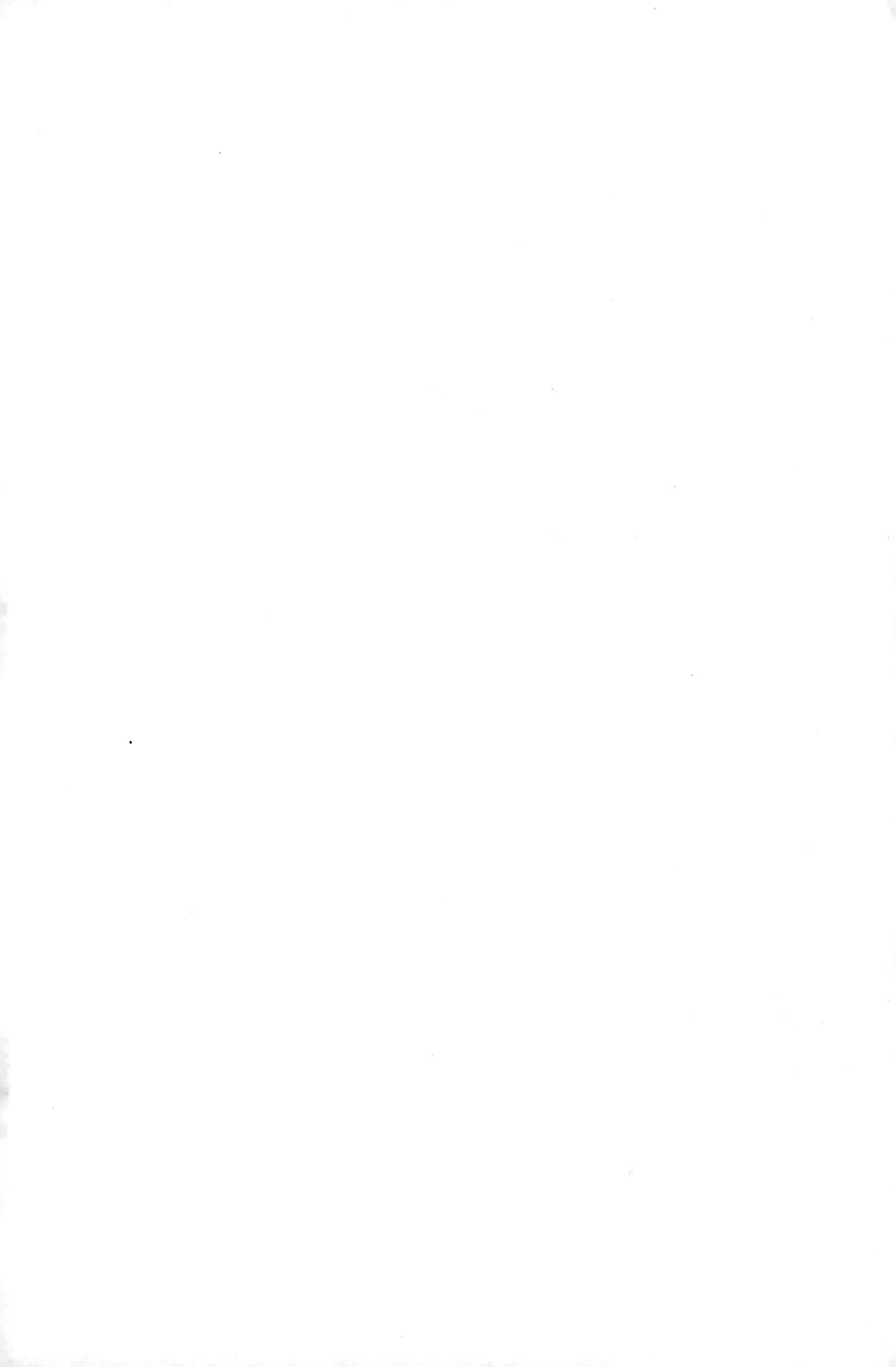

Lightning Source UK Ltd.
Milton Keynes UK
UKHW05f1821060818
326846UK00011B/574/P